John Goodale Briante

The old root and herb doctor

Or, the Indian method of healing

John Goodale Briante

The old root and herb doctor
Or, the Indian method of healing

ISBN/EAN: 9783742830500

Manufactured in Europe, USA, Canada, Australia, Japa

Cover: Foto ©Lupo / pixelio.de

Manufactured and distributed by brebook publishing software (www.brebook.com)

John Goodale Briante

The old root and herb doctor

THE OLD

Root and Herb Doctor,

OR THE

INDIAN METHOD OF HEALING.

BY

DR. JOHN GOODALE BRIANTE,

For many years with the St. Francis Tribe of Indians, at Green Bay; also, for several years with the Pottawattamies and other Tribes.

CONTAINING

Directions for preparing and using their most valuable Remedies, as used by him, in his extensive practice throughout the Eastern and Middle States.

CLAREMONT, N. H.
GRANITE BOOK COMPANY.
1870.

PREFACE.

In preparing this little volume, the Author has labored more to produce something which shall be useful, than he has to issue an elaborate work, which will bear criticism.

The Remedies given may be relied upon, and are the result of a long and careful study of the system followed by the natives of this country, whose singular success in the treatment of disease is well known; and are the same used by the Doctor, during a successful practice of thirty years.

If the directions here laid down are carefully followed it will, in many cases, save the expense and trouble of calling upon the family physician and prove of the greatest value at times when his attendance cannot be procured.

The Doctor has been assisted in the preparation of this work by several friends whose labors have added materially to the value of the work.

CONTENTS.

Alterative Syrup,..18
Anti-Bilious Bitters,...27, 28
Asthma,...27, 53
Astringent Pills,..58
Astringent Injection,...58
Balsam,..43, 49
Blackberry Cordial,..52
Bleeding Piles,..32
Boils,..38
Rroken Breast,..36
Burns and Scalds,..21, 29
Canadian Liniment,..40
Cancer Cure,..30
Canker,...31
Catarrh,..39
Chilblains,..37, 47, 62
Cholera Cordial,..51
Cholera Morbus,..46
Cold in the Head,...31, 42
Cologne Water,...88
Composition,..48
Consumption,...33
Corns,...28, 45, 52

CONTENTS. v

Cosmetic,	54
Costiveness,	87
Cough,	31
Cough Mixture,	26, 47
Cough Remedy,	22
Deafness,	38
Diabetes,	35
Diarrhœa,	25
Directions,	17
Dropsy,	29
Dysentery,	19, 43, 45, 49
Dyspepsia,	34
Dyspeptic Bitters,	21
Eyes,	31
Felon,	44
Fever Sores,	36
Freckle Wash,	53
Gall Ointment,	62
Gravel	41
Green Bay Salve,	35
Headache Lotion,	52
Hemorrhoids,	59
Hiccough,	24
Infusions,	89
Itch Ointment,	51
Jaundice,	23, 50
Kidneys,	43, 40
Leucorrhœa,	54
Liniment,	42, 50
Liniment for Neuralgia,	87
Lip Salve,	53

CONTENTS.

Liver Complaint,	29
Materia Medica,	90
Measles,	22
Metea's Healing Salve,	42
Mothers Cordial,	20
Mucilages,	88
Mustard Emetic,	87
Old Sores,	36
Piles,	22, 24
Pills, for Neuralgia,	87
Poisons,	63
Roots and Herbs,	17
Rheumatism,	28, 34
Rules of Health,	11
Salve,	44
Scarlet Fever,	38
Sore Stomach,	44
Species of Oil,	28
Spirits of Lavender,	48
Stiff Joints,	39
Swelling,	49
Strengthening Mixture,	57
Table,	14
Tape Worm,	31, 40
Tinctures,	89
Tonic Bitters,	33, 89
Toothache,	47
Tooth Powder,	88
Whooping Cough,	32, 39, 53, 45
Wind Colic,	38
Worms,	32, 37

CONTENTS.

Yellow Dock Ointment, ... 22

POISONS AND THEIR ANTIDOTES.

Alcohol, ... 63
Ammonia, ... 64
Aquafortis, ... 64
Arsenic, ... 65
Bismuth, ... 65
Blistering Flies, ... 66
Blue Vitriol, ... 66
Carbonic Acid Gas, ... 67
Cobalt, ... 67
Corrosive Sublimate, ... 68
Deadly Nightshade, ... 68
Fools Parsley, ... 69
Fox Glove, ... 69
Funguses, ... 70
Hellebore, ... 70
Hemlock, ... 71
Henbane, ... 71
Lime, ... 72
Lunar Caustic, ... 72
Meadow Saffron, ... 72
Monks Hood, ... 73
Mountain Laurel, ... 73
Muriatic Acid, ... 74
Muriate of Barytes, ... 74
Muriate of Tin, ... 75
Nitre, ... 75
Nitrate of Silver, ... 76
Nitric Acid, ... 76
Nux Vomica, ... 76

Oil of Cedar,	76
Oil of Rue,	77
Oil of Savin	77
Oil of Tansy,	78
Oil of Tar,	78
Oil of Vitriol,	78
Opium,	79
Oxalic Acid,	80
Phosphorus,	80
Poppies,	81
Potash,	81
Poison Ivy,	41
Poison Dogwood,	41
Prussic Acid,	81
Salt of Sorrel,	82
Stramonium,	82
Strychnia,	82
Sulphate of Copper,	82
Sulphate of Zinc,	82
Sulphuric Acid,	82
Sugar of Lead,	82
Tartar Emetic,	83
Thorn Apple,	83
Tobacco,	84
Verdigris,	84
White Vitriol,	84
White Lead,	84
Wolf's Bane,	86

THE OLD

ROOT AND HERB DOCTOR.

INTRODUCTORY REMARKS.

All men ought to be acquainted with the medicinal qualities of Roots and Herbs; for a knowledge of medicine is the companion of wisdom.

Whoever breaks away from the unchanging laws of nature, and uses those medicines never designed by nature to cure the sick, will find, in the end, that the laws which govern the natural, as well as those which govern the moral world, never change.

"Nature's wants, both in sickness and health, are few and easily supplied. The vegetable remedies which the God of nature has spread out with such richness and profusion over every hill and dale, and field and forest will supersede the use of minerals. The voice of nature speaks everywhere, in language that must be understood by all who hearken to her instructions." The whole surface of the earth, wherever designed for the abode of man, is but one continued apothecary shop. Notwithstanding this, people will shut their eyes, and take upon trust everything that is administered to them by any pretender to medicine, without asking him a reason for any part of his conduct.

Any man can tell when a medicine gives him relief, as well as a physician, and if he only knows the name and dose of the medicine, and the name of the disease he is enabled in many cases to defend himself from imposition.

At the present day, people have become so accustomed to patronizing Quack Doctors and Patent Medicines, that it has become proverbial that it is easier to cheat a man out of his life, than out of a dollar. This book is designed to meet the wants of the class referred to above, and is not the production of one who has a new system to introduce, or a remedy for all aches and pains to sell, but gives advice, founded on common sense, and Nature furnishes the remedy.

GENERAL RULES OF HEALTH.

There is no doubt that more people are injured by eating too much, than by any other cause; in fact, there are but few persons who do not, at times, indulge their appetites beyond what is good for them and overload their stomachs. If this is allowed to become a habit, it will soon produce a derangement of the whole system.

When a person feels uncomfortable by reason of overeating, let him abstain from one or two meals and he will find relief, and his system will be in a much better condition than it would be if he should dose himself with medicine. "Nature has resources within herself to restore the body to healthy action if the stomach is permitted to remain in a state of rest.

There are various opinions in regard to eating meat, but it is well known that the Indians used but little vegetable food, and the small amount which they made use of, was very different from that used by us, and was prepared in the simplest manner.

Food taken between meals, in any quantity, is but a source of irritation to the stomach, and becomes the object of a wearing, unnatural effort on the part of this organ, to effect its digestion. Now it is not the quantity of material that is productive of injury but it is the continual unrelaxing labor that is exacted of the stomach, keeping it constantly at work digesting these morsels, without proper intervals of rest and recuperation.

It is obvious that articles of food repugnant to the stomach, and consequently to the mind, will retard digestion, and induce disease.

Articles of diet, in themselves, whether vegetable or animal, have no part in causing sickness, unless they disagree with the stomach, provided they are properly cooked and eaten, in reasonable quantities, at proper hours. It is from their abuse that evils arise, and to decide what one should eat to promote health, we would say, choose those kinds of food that best suit your taste, and digestion, but do not hasten your death by dieting improperly or eating at improper hours.

Persons should never drink excessively during

meals; it is better not to drink at all, for it is a fact that the Indians seldom, if ever, partook of any liquid at that time. It is very important, also, *what* we drink, for in the days of adulteration, we never know what we buy—Tea and Coffee are both difficult to procure in a state of purity; we mean, of course, *ground* coffee—and our advice is, if it is to be used, buy it in the raw state. In regard to the article of Tea, we would say, there is a perfect substitute for it. Sage tea is excellent to correct the deranged secretions, and to promote health, and its use is urged frequently in the family in preference to some of the black adulterated teas purchased at our stores. Experience teaches that the stomach requires some gentle bitter to keep the bile in a healty condition, and in sage tea, if people would only drink it occasionally, as a substitute for the various kinds of teas, they would find that it would go far towards restoring the nerves and the mind to a healthful condition.

It is very important that a person should be regular at meals—have them at stated times and not eat between them; eat slowly and masticate the food properly, avoid a variety of kinds—make his meal principally of *one* kind of food, and that prepared in a simple manner; and not eat highly seasoned food nor any greasy substances.

If you feel a little unwell, do not take medicine, but abstain from hearty food and allow the system to rest for a day or two.

Never sit down in a perspiration, without putting on more clothing, and never sit in a draft under any circumstances. Keep the feet warm and dry, at all times, if possible, and never go to bed with cold feet; if there is no fire at hand, rub them till they are warm.

TABLE SHOWING THE MEAN TIME OF DIGESTION OF THE DIFFERENT ARTICLES OF FOOD.

		H. M.
Rice.	Boiled,	1.00
Sago,	"	1.45
Tapioca,	"	2.00
Tripe,	"	1.00
Turkey,	Roasted,	2.30
Goose,	"	2.30

Pig,	Roasted,	2.30
Liver,	Broiled,	2.00
Lamb,	"	2.30
Chicken,	"	2.45
Eggs,	Hard boiled,	3.30
Eggs,	Soft boiled,	3.00
Custard,	Baked,	2.45
Codfish, dry,	Boiled,	2.00
Trout, fresh,	"	1.30
Oysters,	Raw,	2.55
Oysters,	Stewed,	3.30
Beef,	Roasted,	3.30
Beef Steak,	Broiled,	3.00
Pork Steak,	"	3.15
Pork,	Roasted,	5.15
Mutton,	"	3.15
Mutton,	Broiled,	3.00
Veal,	"	4.00
Fowls,	Roasted,	4.00
Soup, beef,	Boiled,	4.00
Corn & Beans,	"	3.45
Sausage,	Fried,	3.20
Apples,	Raw,	2.50

Potatoes,	Boiled,	3.30
Potatoes,	Roasted,	2.30
Cabbage,	Boiled,	.4,30
Bread, wheat,		3.30
Bread, corn,		3.15

The following table shows the amount of nourishment in different articles of food, as ascertained by experiment:

100 parts of Bread contain 80 of nourishment
" " " Beans " 86 " "
" " " Rice " 90 " "
" " " Wheat " 85 " "
" " " Rye " 80 " "
" " " Meat, average, 35 " "
" " " Potatoes " 25 " "
" " " Carrots " 14 " "
" " " Beets " 14 " "
" " " Turnips " 8 " "
" " " Cabbage " 7 " "
" " " Greens " 6 " "

TIME FOR COLLECTING ROOTS AND HERBS.

The best time to collect roots is late in the Fall, after the tops have died, or else in the Spring before they have started up.

Herbs should be gathered when in full blossom, and should be dried in the shade. After they are well dried, they should be packed in something tight, as they will lose strength if exposed to the air.

DIRECTIONS.

It is not possible to lay down any rule that will be a guide, in regard to doses of medicine in all cases. We can only show what is an ordinary portion in common cases, and the person who administers the medicine should exercise judgment as to the proper quantity to be given.

Always ascertain how medicine operates with the sick person, whether easy or not, and make the dose accordingly.

For a general rule, persons require a full dose at twenty, though women a little less than men. It is very important that there be a competent nurse, but no matter how well qualified that person may be, some friend or relative should always be in attendance.

The following household implements are frequently used for the sake of convenience, and for want of accurate measures. Custom has attached to each the following proportions:

A Pint contains sixteen ounces.
A Tea-cup contains a gill or four fluid ounces.
A Wine-glass contains two ounces.
A Table-spoon contains one half an ounce.
A Dessert-spoon contains one quarter of an ounce.
A Tea-spoon contains sixty drops.
Four Tea-spoonfuls equal one Table-spoonful.

In Dry Measure, where a spoon or spoonful is mentioned, the design is, that the spoon should be taken up moderately rounding, unless otherwise mentioned.

ALTERATIVE SYRUP.

Take three pounds of Sarsaparilla, two pounds of Guaiacum shavings, half a pound of Sassafras root, one pound Elder flowers, one pound Black Alder buds, one pound Burdock seeds. Boil these together for three hours, turn off the liquor, and fill up again with water: boil again for the same length of time, put it together and boil down to ten or twelve quarts, or thereabouts. Add eight pounds of loaf sugar, put in a few eggs, beat them up, and boil till no scum rises.

This makes a very excellent medicine which should be prepared and kept in every family.

It is good in cases of Rheumatism, Inflammation of the Liver, Scrofula, Ulcers, Cutaneous Diseases, and White Swellings. If this syrup is made when the weather is warm, you must add a quart of Alcohol, that it may not sour. The DOSE is *two-thirds of a wineglass*, three times a day.

DYSENTERY.

This disease is distinguished from diarrhœa by an acute pain in the bowels, and by the discharge of bloody matter. It is most prevalent in the Spring and Fall. It is frequently caused by night air, unwholesome air, bad water, taking off flannels, wet clothes &c.

The symptoms are griping pain in the bowels; inclination to go to stool; bloody, slimy discharges, and it is often attended with chills and quickening of the pulse.

It may be cured, in the first stages, by giving boiled milk, thickened with flour. If this should check the disease too suddenly, give half a teaspoonful of rhubarb, which will physic gently, and after two hours give half a pint of strong thoroughwort tea.

An Indian, on the coast of Labrador, once cured the son of a sea captain by giving him a strong decoction, made by boiling a quantity of double spruce tops, and afterwards giving a gentle portion of physic.

MOTHER'S CORDIAL.

Take half a pound of Squaw Root, (Black Snake-root) pour three pints of boiling water on it, steep gently four or five hours, to about a quart, add two teaspoonfuls of the flour of Slippery Elm, and one pound of loaf sugar.

For Heart-burn and Sickness at the Stomach take

a *tumbler full* in the course of the day. Women, who, under certain circumstances, are troubled in this way, will generally find it a great relief. Persons who are apt to vomit up their food will find it a good preventive.

DYSPEPTIC BITTERS.

Take four ounces of Golden Seal, two ounces of Bitter Root, four ounces of Poplar bark, four ounces of Peach-meats: add two quarts of Gin and two quarts of water. Take *two thirds of a wine-glass*, before eating. It is very good in cases of Dyspepsia, and weakness of the stomach. In cases where food produces distress, it should be taken *after* eating

BURNS AND SCALDS.

In a case of severe burn, a poultice should be used made of the flour of Slippery Elm, and sweet oil. This will be found a great relief. Another very good remedy is a paste made of flour and water, spread on a cloth, which should be changed as often as it gets dry. Above all things, keep the parts from the air.

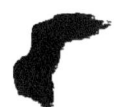

COUGH REMEDY.

Take one ounce of Elecampane, half an ounce of Hoarhound, an ounce and a half of Liquorice root, two ounces of Sulphur. Pulverize them, and add honey. Take a *tea-spoonful*, at intervals, as needful.

YELLOW DOCK OINTMENT.

Take common Yellow Dock, pour cream over it and simmer together gently. It makes a good ointment which will be found very cooling in cases of humors.

PILE OINTMENT.

Take a handful of Jimson leaves and the same quantity of Parsley, and stew them in a pound of lard.

MEASLES.

The first appearances of Measles are small eruptions upon the face and body, more particularly the face and neck, which do not tend to produce pus. These spots afterward run together and form red streaks, and produce some swelling in the face.—Measles is a contagious disease, but persons seldom have it a second time. In many respects it resembles

Small Pox, and the general course of treatment should be about the same. The patient shouid be kept in the house, and the rooms warm at all times, as sudden changes are apt to cause the measles to strike in. A strong tea, made of Saffron and Snakeroot, Pennyroyal or Mayweed should be used freely After the measles has fairly turned, give a good portion of physic. In most cases, but little medicine is needed, for with a little assistance, nature will do the work.

JAUNDICE.

This disease is first observable in the eye, which has a yellow appearance, and afterwards the whole skin takes the same hue; the urine is also of the same saffron hue and will dye a white cloth if wet with it. The following has proved very successful in many cases.

Take equal parts of Soot and Saffron; tie them up in a cloth to the size of half a hen's egg, let it lie in a glass of water over night, in the morning put the yolk of an egg, beaten, into this water and drink it. Do this three mornings, then skip three, until nine doses have been taken.

HICCOUGH.

When it arises from the use of food that is hard of digestion, Wine or any spiritous liquors may be used; sometimes a little Vinegar will answer the purpose. If poison be the cause, take plenty of Oil and Milk. When it proceeds from Inflammation of the stomach, cooling driuks should be taken. Hops and Wormwood, simmered in vinegar should be applied to the Stomach.

PILES.

This disease is caused by a painful swelling of the Intestinal vessels. When they discharge no blood, they are called Blind Piles; but when they discharge blood, they are called Bleeding Piles. The pi es are brought on by various causes; more frequently by much sitting, whether at work or riding. Some constitutions are more inclined to this disease than others, and as soon as a person finds that it is coming on, he should change his business, if it be a sedentary one. He should go to stool at the same hour every day, and keep his bowels open with gentle purgatives, and anoint the parts with Sweet oil and flour of Hemlock bark, or take powdered Opium, and powdered Resin, and Tallow, one ounce each, and anoint. Another remedy is a strong tea, made of the wild Swamp Currant root, drinking it for a few days only. When falling of the bowels takes place, take White Oak bark, Witch Hazel bark, and Upland Sumac, equal parts, make a decoction, add a tea-spoonful of pulverized Alum to every pint, and apply from time to time. Let the bowels be kept open with Yellow Dock, and avoid high living.

DIARRHŒA.

This is not a disease in all cases, but it is nature trying to get rid of disease. It should not be checked unless it produces weakness.

It is said that about five hundred of the Oneida tribe of Indians were attacked by this disease at one time, and were all cured by the use of blackberry root, whilst many of their white neighbors died of the same disorder.

When this disease is brought on by ong use of Calomel, take Boxwood, Black Cherry and Prickly Ash barks with Dandelion root—each, two ounces:

Butternut bark, one ounce: boil thoroughly, strain and boil down to one quart, add two pounds loaf sugar, one gill alcohol and take a *wine-glassful* from three to five times daily.

Sumac bobs, steeped and sweetened with loaf sugar have been very valuable in this disease, adding, in severe cases, a tea-spoonful of pulverized alum to one pint of the tea.

Dose: *from a tea to a table-spoonful*, according to the age of the child.

COUGH MIXTURE.

Take one ounce of Blood Root, one ounce of Senna leaves, one ounce of Anise Seed, one ounce of Senega Root; boil these together in one quart of water until half evaporated, then strain it and add four ounces of loaf sugar. Dose: one *tea-spoonful*, three times a day. This is one of the best remedies ever used by any one, and should be kept in every family where there are children.

COUGH MIXTURE.

Take two ounces Tincture of Blood Root, one ounce Elixir Asthmatic, two ounces Hive Syrup;

mix thoroughly and give *one tea-spoonful* two or three times a day. The above ingredients can be obtained at any Drug Store.

REMEDY FOR ASTHMA.

Take one half ounce Elecampane root, pulverized, one half ounce of Flos Sulphur, four scruples of Belladonna leaves, pulverized, one Drachm of Senega root; Mix them well and divide into ninety powders, one of which is to be taken three times a day.

RHEUMATIC LINIMENT.

Take one ounce Tincture of Camphor, two ounces Tincture of Aconite, one half ounce Cayenne, two and one half Drachms Aqua Ammonia, mix thoroughly and apply to the part affected.

ANTI-BILIOUS BITTERS.

Take one and one half ounce of Mandrake, one ounce of Gentian, one ounce of Yellow Dock root, one ounce of Wild Cherry bark and four pints of diluted Alcohol; put the whole into a large bottle and let it stand forty-eight hours, then take one table-spoonful of the mixture three times a day.

ANTI-BILIOUS BITTERS.

Take one ounce of Yellow Dock root, one ounce of Dandelion root, one ounce of Mandrake, one ounce of Gentian, one ounce of Serpentaria, one ounce of Sassafras bark, and put the whole into four pints of diluted Alcohol, and let it stand forty-eight hours. DOSE. Give *one or two table-spoonfuls*, according to the patient, and the stage of the disease.

RHEUMATISM.

SPECIES OF OIL.

Take 1 pint Skunk's oil, 1 pint Spirits of Turpentine, 1 pint Oil of Spike, 2 ounces Oil of Vitriol. Mix these and let the mixture settle, and it will be very clear. Rub it on the places where the lameness seems to be, *very thoroughly.*

Keep the mixture in a bottle, well corked, and shake it well before using. The Vitriol should be handled with great care.

CORNS.

Apply the "specie of oil" to the corn, once a day.

The Oil of Spike can be made by placing a quantity of Fish Worms in a bottle, and hanging it in the sun until they are dissolved.

LIVER COMPLAINT.

Take the root of Man of the Earth, and pulverize, then to 4 spoonfuls of it add one-half pound Jalap root; Pipsissewa herb, 2 pounds; Snake-root, 4 ounces; Saffron, 3 ounces. For an adult, *a wineglassful*, three times a day, before eating.

SALVE FOR BURNS.

Mix raw potato, scraped, with Flaxseed, and bind it on the burnt part: afterward, use an ointment made of Soot, from the stovepipe, and fresh lard, simmered together; spread it on a cloth and lay it on the sore.

DROPSY.

Take blue or white Vervain, steep it and drink the decoction freely—this will carry away the water. Then give a Syrup made of the following:

Three pounds Sweet Fern, 2 ounces Pulsely, Yellow Dock; ½ pound, Pipsissewa or Wintergreen,

2 pounds: white Snake-root, ¼ pound, or of the herb, 1½ pounds; Bitter Sweet, ¼ pound. Steep together, and, for an adult, give a *wine-glassful*, sweetened, 3 times a day or 5 times if it is a severe case. The above quantities are for one gallon, and it should be kept in a cool place.

CANCER CURE.

Take "King of all Poison," pound up, and pulverize it, bind it on the Cancer, and it will take out the inflammation. Then use a wash made as follows: take hard-wood ashes, leach them, and boil down the liquor till it is very strong.

Apply this twice a day with a swab, to kill the Cancer. A Syrup should be taken, made of the following articles,—it is called Was-a-mo-s medicine.

One-pound Spikenard Root, 3 pounds Sweet Fern Root; ½ pound Yellow Dock Root: ½ pound Elecampane root, 1½ pound White Vervain herb, 1½ pounds Pigeon Cherry bark, 1½ pounds White Pine bark, ½ pound Sweet Sicily, ½ pound Blood Root. Dose, *a wine-glassful*, three times a day, using reason about giving, according to health, age, &c. This Syrup is an excellent medicine in all cases of Slow Fever, Bilious complaints, Costiveness, &c., decreasing the dose as may be thought necessary.

INFLAMMATION OF THE EYES.

Take "King of all Poison,"—which may be found on white oak land—pound it up and pulverize it and bind it on the eyes, over night.

COLD IN THE HEAD.

Take either Pipsissewa or Hoarhound, steep it and drink freely before going to bed.

CANKER IN THE MOUTH.

Take Balmonia, or Snake's Head, steep it strong and wash the mouth thoroughly with the liquor.

TAPE-WORMS.

Take "Man of the Earth" root, steep it and give very strong. This has proved very effectual.

COUGH.

Take 1 pound of Cumfrey, 1 pound of Spikenard, 1 pound Motherwort, ½ pound Oak of Jerusalem, ½ pound Balmonia, steep them together and give a *wine-glassful*, 3 times a day before eating. A half pound Hoarhound may be used in place of the Oak of Jerusalem.

BLEEDING PILES.

Take 1 pound of Polly Flowers, steep them and strain the decoction; give 3 *tea-spoonfuls*, three times a day, before eating.

WORMS IN CHILDREN.

Take the bark of Spotted Alder, or Witch Hazel and steep it in water, over a slow fire, till the liquid is very strong.

Dose, a *table-spoonful*, three times a day, for a child a year old.

To prevent worms, let children eat Onions freely, either raw or cooked.

REMEDY FOR WHOOPING COUGH.

Take a quarter of a pound of Elecampane root, ground fine, mix with half a pint of strained Honey and half a pint of water—put them in a stone jar and place it in the oven with half the heat required to bake bread, let it remain till as thick as Honey. Dose for a child; *one tea-spoonful* before eating, for an adult, double that quantity.

BRIANTE'S TONIC BITTERS.

Take one pound of Wild Cherry bark, and boil in a quart of water till reduced to a pint, sweeten and add one gill of Spirit to preserve it.

Dose, a *wine-glassful* three times a day, on an empty stomach.

HOARSENESS AND SORE THROAT.

Take a quantity of Spikenard root, bruise it and steep in a teapot, using water and two thirds as much spirits, let it cool a little, then inhale the steam through the nose. It will give great relief and take away the soreness.

CONSUMPTION.

Take Tamarack bark, without rossing, 1 peck; Spikenard root, ½ pound, Dandelion root, ¼ pound; Hops 2 ounces. Boil these together long enough to extract the strength, in two or three gallons of water —when it is lukewarm, put in 3 pounds of Honey, and

3 pints of good Brandy. Dose: a *wine-glass* three times a day before eating. It is not expected that all cases of Consumption can be cured, but many cases, *called* Consumption, have been cured by the use of this Syrup, and it is certainly worth a trial, and if the disease is not inherited there is great hope.

DYSPEPSIA.

Take Chamomile flowers, Scullcap, Thoroughwort—each, 2 pounds; 1 pound each of Hops, Spearmint, bark of Sassafras root, Juniper berries, Gentian root, Yellow Dock root and Mandrake; ½ pound Anise seed; 1 oz. Cayenne. Steep and strain and to five parts of the liquor add one of Spirit.

Dose, *one great spoonful*, three times a day, before eating. This is an excellent remedy for nervous diseases and is very strengthening.

RHEUMATISM.

The following is used with great success by the Green Bay Indians:

Wahoo, bark of the root, 1 ounce; Blood root, 1 ounce, Black Cohosh 2 ounces, Swamp Hellebore

½ ounce, Prickly Ash bark 1 ounce, Poke root cut fine 1 ounce, Rye Whisky 1 quart. Let it stand a few days before using.

DOSE: *one tea-spoonful* every 3 or 4 hours, increasing the dose as the stomach will bear it.

DIABETIS.

Take "Queen of the Meadows" root, steep it and drink freely before eating. Another remedy is a Syrup made of equal parts of Yarrow and common Plantain.

BRONCHITIS.

Take Blue or White Vervain, steep and give a wine-glass full three times a day. Rub the neck and stomach with "Specie of Oil." (See Receipt.)

GREEN BAY SALVE.

Beeswax 2 pounds, Mutton Tallow 2 pounds, White Pine Turpentine 1 pint, 1 oz. Verdigris, 1 pint old Rum, simmer these together, except the Verdigris, which should not be put in until the rest are mixed. Be careful not to burn the mixture. Let it settle and take the bottom for the Salve. This will be found very good to heal old sores, Fever sores, fresh Cuts, Wounds and Bruises of every kind.

FEVER SORES.

If there is inflammation put on a poultice made of White Beans, parboiled and mashed, or of Sweet Pumpkins stewed and sifted, then, to heal it, use the Green Bay Salve. The system should be cleansed by taking "Was-a-mo-s Medicine" three times a day before eating,—if this should not operate. increase the Dose.

If it is an old sore and refuses to heal, use the Indian Cancer Cure to kill it.

OLD SORES.

Take the root of the "Indian Wickerby" and make a poultice of it. It will be found one of the best things for Old Sores or Inflammation.

BROKEN BREAST.

Take Pennyroyal root and Lovage root, pound them up together, and make a poultice,—bind it on the breast. Another remedy is green Burdock leaves, which should be placed on the stove and wilted, after which lay them on and cover with a warm cloth, until it sweats the part. Perhaps the best remedy is White Beans, which should be par-boiled soft, and then mashed, and made into a poultice, which should be put on cold.

PILES.

Take an old Boot and burn it to a crisp, pulverize and pass it through a sieve, mix with fresh Lard. Anoint the parts several times a day, using the Syrup for Bleeding Piles.

WORMS.

Take Poplar bark, pulverize it and mix with Molasses. Dose, *a tea-spoonful twice a day before eating*, or steep the bark and give three tea-spoonfuls a day before eating.

SORE LIPS, CHAPPED HANDS, CHILBLAINS.

Take Golden Thread or Mouth root—as it is called by the Indians—and Chamomile, and simmer together in Hog's Lard; apply freely, rubbing it in well.

DEAFNESS.

Take a small quantity of good Ginger root, and 3 ounces fresh Butter, simmer together. Strain it clean, and drop a small quantity into the ear once a day, say 3 drops, then put in a piece of cotton, keep it there.

FOR BOILS.

Take a good sized Onion, roast it in the ashes,—mash it and put it on for a poultice. It will bring it to a head very soon.

The juice of an Onion, sweetened with Sugar, is very good for a Cold or Hoarseness.

WIND COLIC.

Take a handful of Pennyroyal, steep it, making a strong tea, and drink every fifteen minutes.

SCARLET FEVER.

Every person sick with this disease should have a drink made of the following; Take equal parts of Cleavers, and Elder blows, put them in warm water and let them stand three hours when cold: it may be taken freely.

WHOOPING COUGH.

Take two ounces Wild Snow Ball bark, and steep it in a quart of water.

Dose, *one table-spoonful, three times a day.*

CATARRH.

Take Red Clover blossoms, perhaps a double handful, put them in a pint and a half of water and steep very strong, strain off the liquor and boil it down very thick, till it is like wax, let it cool, then dry it in the sun or an oven till it is hard, then pound it very fine and use it for snuff.

This has cured many persons.

OINTMENT FOR STIFF JOINTS.

Take equal parts of Bitter-Sweet bark, Purple Archangel, Chamomile and Meadow Fern burrs. Crowd them tightly into a vessel and cover them with Goose Oil. Simmer together slowly for eight hours, keeping it well covered. Strain off the mixture, and, after it has stood an hour, add an ounce of Spearmint Oil. This should be kept in a tight bottle.

CANADIAN LINIMENT.

Take equal parts of Stramonium leaves, High Mallows, and House Leeks, put them all into a vessel with a sufficient quantity of water and boil till quite strong, then add one quart of Sweet Cream and simmer it down over a slow fire until the water has all disappeared, then strain it and keep in a bottle, closely corked.

KIDNEY COMPLAINT.

Take two handfuls of blue Vervain and steep it in one quart of water, strain it and add one pound of Honey. Drink a tumblerful three times a day. It will be found a valuable remedy.

BRIANTE'S STRENGTHENING PLASTER.

Take one pound and a half of Pitch Pine, two ounces of Beeswax, two ounces of Hemlock Gum, two ounces of fresh Lard. Melt these and add half a gill of Brandy and a quarter of an ounce of Sweet Oil and the same of Sassafras oil and Camphor. When these articles are well mixed, pour them into a pail of cold water and work them with the hands. In the Summer, Resin may be used instead of Pitch Pine.

Spread this compound on soft leather, and apply to the part affected.

A SIMPLE REMEDY FOR LIVER COMPLAINT.

Take one ounce of Wormwood, put it in a bottle containing one pint of good Gin. Let it stand over night, and take one table-spoonful three times a day.

IVY OR DOGWOOD POISON.

Take equal quantities of Lobelia and Elm bark and make a poultice by adding a little weak Lye,—bind this on the part, and renew as often as it dries.

GRAVEL.

Take Dwarf Elder bark, Queen of the Meadow root, Marshmallow root and trailing Arbutus, half an ounce of each, pound them up and add a pint of hot water and three gills of Holland Gin; steep it in a covered kettle, then strain it and add a little honey.

BRIANTE'S LINIMENT.

Take one Gill Spirits Turpentine, two ounces Camphor Gum, one half ounce Spirits Hartshorn, two ounces Origanum, two ounces Wormwood, half pint, each Sweet Oil and Alcohol. Put the whole into a large bottle, and shake until well mixed.

This mixture is very good for Rheumatism, or lameness of any kind.

TO BREAK UP A COLD IN THE HEAD.

Take a small quantity of Wormwood, and make a strong tea of it, sweeten well with sugar and take a tumbler full hot, after getting into bed, cover up warm, and, if it is cold weather, hot stones should be placed at the feet. This is a sure remedy.

METEA'S HEALING SALVE.

Take two ounces of Beeswax and two ounces of Burgundy Pitch, or White Pine Pitch, and two ounces of Sweet Oil. Melt them well together, stirring them well till cold.

This will be found an excellent preparation for healing old sores, burns, cuts, &c.

INFLAMMATION OF THE KIDNEYS.

Take two and a half ounces of Cleavers (the herb) and put it in one quart of warm water,—let it stand three hours. Take a tumbler full three times a day.

INDIAN HEALING BALSAM.

Take white Resin, 3 pounds; melt it and add 1½ pints Turpentine, then put in 4 oz. Fir Balsam, 1 oz. Balsam of Tolu, 1 oz. Oil of Hemlock, 1 oz. of Oil of Origanum, 4 oz. strained Honey, and shake well together.

Dose, 10 *drops*, and, for a child, give half that quantity or less as the stomach may bear it. This will also be found to give relief in diseases of the kidneys.

FOR DYSENTERY.

Take a couple of handfuls of Indian Corn and roast it in a kettle the same as for Coffee, then pour boiling water on it and let it stand three hours, after which drink freely, clear, three or four times a day.

SALVE.

Take 4 pounds Resin, ½ pound White Pine Pitch, ¼ pound of Beeswax, ¼ pound Mutton Tallow, ½ oz. Fir Balsam, 1 oz., Sweet Oil, ¼ pint Alcohol, mix the same as for any other Salve.

CURE FOR FELON.

Take the root of Poke and roast it in the ashes until it is soft, then mash it and bind it on as a poultice. It is a sure cure if taken in season.

ANOTHER CURE FOR FELON.

Take common rock Salt, such as is used for salting meat, dry it in an oven, then pound it up fine and mix with Spirits of Turpentine equal parts; spread it on a cloth and bind on the sore, and as soon as it gets dry, put on more. This will kill a Felon in twenty-four hours.

FOR SORE STOMACH.

Take the Indian Turnip, which may be found in nearly all forests; dry it and pulverize fine, take half a *tea-spoonful* in molasses on going to bed. The soreness will be gone after two or three doses.

DYSENTERY.

Take equal parts of the bark of Spruce root, Strawberry leaves and Cumfrey root. Boil an ounce of the compound, or more if dry, in a pint of milk, take it freely with Crackers if desired.

CURE FOR CORNS.

Make one ounce of Gum Ammoniac, one ounce Yellow Wax and three drachms of Verdigris;— melt them together and spread the composition on soft leather. Cut away the corn as much as you can and apply the Plaster, and renew, every week, until cured.

CEPHALIC SNUFF.

Take three parts of Asarbacca leaves dried; one part of Marjoram; one part Lavender flowers; and reduce them to a fine powder;—use if for a Snuff.

FOR WHOOPING COUGH.

Take three ounces of Chesnut leaves, and boil in a pint of water for a short time only, then pour the whole into a teapot, without straining, and drink often, especially at bed-time, either cold or warm, with or without sugar.

FOR LIVER COMPLAINT.

Take "Snake's Head," and fill a quart bottle ½ full with the leaves, and then fill up with good Cider,— let it stand over night, then drink two or three times a day freely. The leaves will be strong enough to fill up a second time.

CHOLERA MORBUS.

Take two ounces of the leaves of the Bean plant and put them in a pint of cold water and let them stand an hour.

Give *two table-spoonfuls*, each hour until relief is experienced.

INDIAN REMEDY FOR TAPE-WORM.

Take a quantity of Sweet Fern; put it in three pints of water, and boil it down, making a strong decoction.

Dose: *two thirds of a tumblerful*, three times a day, and on the fifth day take a dose of some kind of physic.

OINTMENT FOR CHILBLAINS.

Take equal parts of Yellow Root, or Gold-thread and common Elder bark,—simmer them together in fresh Lard. No family should be without this ointment.

COUGH MIXTURE.

Take six drachms Tinc. Bloodroot, six drachms Wine of Antimony, six drachms Wine of Ipecac, eight ounces Syrup Tolu, six ounces Mucilage of Gum Arabic, ten grains Sulph. Morphine. Mix these and give *one tea-spoonful* three times a day.

CURE FOR TOOTHACHE.

Wash the mouth thoroughly with a solution of Bi Carbonate of Soda in warm water. Let the gum around the tooth be scarified with a fine lancet, and put a small piece of cotton, moistened with the following preparation, into the cavity of the tooth.

One scruple Tannic Acid, five grains Gum Mastic and two drachms Sulphuric Ether.

This will relieve, in nearly every case.

COMPOSITION.

Take two pounds of Bayberry bark, one pound Hemlock bark, one pound of good Ginger, two ounces of Cayenne, two ounces of Cloves. The whole should be powdered and thoroughly mixed.

Dose: Put a *tea-spoonful* in a cup and pour on boiling water, and drink it as hot as can be borne.

It is of great value in cases of colds and coughs.

COMPOUND SPIRITS OF LAVENDER.

Take seven scruples Oil of Lavender, three and one half scruples Oil Rosemary, one ounce Cinnamon bark, bruised, one ounce Nutmeg, six drachms Red Sanders, six drachms Cloves, one gallon diluted Alcohol. Let the mixture stand ten days and then filter.

This is a very fine compound of Spices and the recipe is given on account of its general use. It is a remedy for gastric uneasiness, nausea, flatulence, and general languor or faintness.

The DOSE is from *thirty drops to a tea-spoonful*, and is most conveniently administered on a lump of sugar.

BALSAM OF WILD CHERRY.

Take two pounds Wild Cherry bark; one ounce Barbadoes Tar; one ounce Ext. Liquorice; two ounces Anise Seed. Boil these in four quarts of water until half evaporated, express and filter it, after which add one ounce of Tinct. Opium.

Dose: *One tea-spoonful*, once or twice a day.

FOR COMMON SWELLING.

Take Tony Weed and pound it so as to mash thoroughly, and bind it upon the part, and it will soon reduce it to its natural size.

It is very valuable in all cases of Rheumatic swelling.

REMEDY FOR DYSENTERY.

Take sixteen grains of Rhubarb; thirty-two grains Sal Tartar, forty-eight grains Prepared Chalk, four drops Oil Spearmint, twenty drops Tinct. Opium, and two fluid ounces of distilled Water.

For a child, the dose is *one tea-spoonful;* for an adult give *one table-spoonful*, sweetened with refined sugar, three or four times a day.

RHEUMATIC LINIMENT.

Take four ounces of Castile Soap, four ounces Oil Origanum, four ounces Tinct. Camphor, four ounces Spirits Ammonia, and two pints Alcohol.

Mix these and rub the part affected, thoroughly, and then cover with flannel.

STRENGTHENING LINIMENT.

Take one ounce Barbadoes Tar, one ounce Balsam of Fir, one ounce Tincture of Opium, three ounces Oil Origanum, four ounces Alcohol.

This should be thoroughly rubbed in, and is a valuable Liniment in cases of lameness or weakness.

JAUNDICE BITTERS.

Take two drachms Myrrh, two drachms Aloes, two drachms Gentian, two drachms Chamomile Flowers, two drachms Galangal, two drachms Orange-peel, one drachm Cardamom Seeds, and two pints diluted Alcohol. Mix the whole and let it stand fourteen days, and then filter.

Dose: *One or two table-spoonfuls*, twice a day.

These Bitters excite the appetite, and invigorate

the powers of digestion, and may be used in all cases of disease, dependent on pure debility of the digestive organs, or requiring a general tonic impression.

CHOLERA CORDIAL.

Take four ounces Tinct. Cayenne; two ounces Myrrh; six fluid drachms Tinct. Opium; three fluid drachms Tinct. Camphor; two and a half fluid drachms Spirits Ammonia.

Dose: *One tea-spoonful,* in a wine-glass of sweetened water, repeated as occasion requires.

The above remedy has long been successfully used in cases of Cholera, Dysentery and Diarrhœa.

ITCH OINTMENT.

Take twelve ounces of fresh Lard, two ounces Red Precipitate, two ounces Burgundy Pitch and two ounces Spirits Turpentine; mix these thoroughly and apply to the affected surface. Another very good Ointment is made of one ounce of powdered White Hellebore root, four ounces of fresh Lard and twelve drops Oil of Lemon, rubbed well together.

TO CURE CORNS.

Take one ounce Nitric Acid, two drachms Dragon's Blood, three drachms Gum Assafœtida, one drachm Lunar Caustic. Apply this with a camel's hair brush, and never afterwards wear tight boots.

HEADACHE LOTION.

Take one ounce Aqua Ammonia, nine ounces Distilled Water, two drachms Chlo. Soda, one half a fluid drachm Spirits Camphor, and a few drops Oil of Roses. In ordinary cases of headache this will relieve.

BLACKBERRY CORDIAL.

Put a large jar of Blackberries into a pot of water, boil them till the juice is out, then strain through a flannel cloth and add Spices, Sugar, Cinnamon and Cloves to the taste. Put it on again and boil fifteen or twenty minutes; then skim and let it cool, and to three quarts of the juice add one quart of the best French Brandy. This makes a splendid cordial for family use.

DAMASK LIP SALVE.

Take eighteen ounces Olive Oil, one pound White Wax, one and a half ounces Spermaceti, one half drachm Oil Rhodium. Mix the whole together over a slow fire, or water bath, and color slightly with a small quantity of Alkanet.

DROPS FOR ASTHMA.

Take two ounces Syrup of Orange Pee, one half ounce Wine of Ipecac, one half drachm Tr. Stramonium, one drachm Tr. Opium.

In severe attacks, give *one tea-spoonful* every hour.

FRECKLE WASH.

Take two ounces Lemon-juice, one half drachm Borate of Soda, powdered, one drachm refined Sugar: mix and let it stand seven days.

FOR WHOOPING COUGH.

Take one drachm Carb. Potass., ten grains of powdered Cochineal, one half pint boiling water, and refined sugar sufficient to form a syrup.

Dose: For an infant, *one tea-spoonful*, three times

a day. In violent cases, the following Liniment should be well rubbed, morning and night, over the whole course of the Spine. One half ounce Aqua Ammonia and one half ounce Oil Amber, mixed.

COSMETIC, MILK OF ROSES.

Take one ounce Oil of Almonds, six grains Sub. Carb. Potass., two drachms Ess. Bergamot, three ounces Rose Water, two drachms Orange-flower water.

This is given for the reason that the use of some such article has become quite common. It is not used by the Indians!

LEUCORRHŒA.

This is the most prevalent of all derangements of the female economy, connected with the uterine system; and from its debilitating effects, induces a train of maladies that tend to embitter personal comfort more than any other human ill. Leucorrhœa consists of a discharge of acid or bland, but variously colored mucus, from the vagina, differing in intensity according to the cause or duration.

It exists with the married and single, with the chaste as well as the unchaste; and therefore the cause of it should be cautiously divined, it being evident that other than sexual indulgences establish this most annoying and distressing affliction.

It may be fairly conceded to be a vitiated secretion, depending upon a weakened state of the local vessels; and, moreover, in particular habits, to a salutary evacuation. On the other hand, it must not be denied that it is oftentimes, the result of sexual intemperance or disease springing from an indiscriminate indulgence in the same. The following may be received as a summary of what occurs, and what should be done for the removal of this disease.

In addition to the discharge, which at one time is scanty, at another profuse, there are usually severe pains in the loins, and the lower part of the abdomen; there is a sense of bearing down, as though the womb were descending, and even protruding. The general health of the patient is disturbed, which is variously apparent, as in loss of appetite, excessive languor, a pale and emaciated look, sleepless nights, dark arcola around the eyes, various hysterical and other nervous affections, and numerous disturbances, indicating a weakened and impaired state of mind and body. Among other causes of the disease beside those alluded to, may be enumerated, irregular living, late hours, mental and bodily fatigue, deficient exercise, impure air, and neglect of personal ablution.

Treatment. In leucorrhœa depending on loss of tone of the secretive vessels of the internal organs of generation, the chief indication is to impart vigor and restore strength, which it is evident depends much upon an avoidance of those causes which originated the disease.

Although leucorrhœa bears a strong resemblance to gonorrhœa, there are points by which to distinguish the one from the other. In gonorrhœa, the discharge is unceasing, but small in quantity, and is usually accompanied by inflammatory symptoms, whereas in leucorrhœa, the discharge is irregular and copious, often coming away in large lumps.

The treatment of leucorrhœa is indicated by the degree of severity present. Where the prominent feature is the discharge, the indication is to increase the action of the absorbents, by restoring the tone of the diseased surface, and at the same time to strengthen the system.

Where the disease is complicated with weakness, and relaxation, astringents should be given by the mouth, and also administered in the form of injections. The alkaline solution of copaiba is very valuable and may be taken twice or thrice daily. It may also be employed as an injection by adding one or two ounces to a pint of water, and a tea-cupful thrown up several times during the day. There are many domestic remedies, which, from their harmless properties, can at least do no injury, if they are not productive of good; as for instance a strong decoction of green Tea, an infusion of white oak bark, or alum water, or diluted Port Wine, all to be used as injections, if it so pleases the patient, may be tried prior to the annexed formulas. The first is a

STRENGTHENING MIXTURE.

Take seven and a half ounces, Infusion of bark, one half drachm diluted Sulp. Acid, two drachms syrup of Orange peel.

Dose: *Three table-spoonfuls*, two or three times a day.

ASTRINGENT PILLS FOR LEUCORRHŒA.

Take one drachm Ext. Peruvian bark, one drachm Gum Kino, one half drachm Alum, one scruple of Nutmeg, Simple syrup sufficient to form the mass. Divide into thirty-six pills.

Dose: *Three pills*, three times a day, to be followed by a tea-cup of lime water.

ANOTHER.—Take thirty grains Alum, one drachm Catechu, five grains Opium, of which make thirty pills.

Dose: Take *three* twice a day.

ASTRINGENT INJECTION.

Take one half ounce compound solution of Alum, and two pints water. This may be used two or three times a day. If it irritates, dilute with water. The following may be used, if desired. One drachm Catechu, one drachm Myrrh, and one half pint Lime-water mixed.

HEMORRHOIDS OR PILES.

As this disease is generally considered to be of a delicate nature, and one about which the afflicted are unwilling to speak, we shall say a few words in regard to them. Piles constitute a disease that may be very slow, or very rapid in its progress. The patient complains of an occasional itching, or soreness at the rectum, after an evacuation—more particularly if subject to constipation, or if he be an irregular liver; when, after a while, he will be surprised on discovering, subsequent to some straining effort, a knot of elastic, but irregularly formed tumors, of about the size of a hazel nut, springing apparently from the rectum, which, in a few days, if they continue, will become sore, and probably be attended with a discharge of blood. Another patient will experience similar symptoms, as regards the pain, swelling, and discharge of blood, except that they will be increased in severity, and be more transitory in their appearance and stay. Upon examination a perceptible difference will be discovered. In the former instance the tumors will be seen to proceed from the outer edge of the rectum, and will be found to be covered with the common skin. This form of the disease is designated, "External Piles." In the latter, the tumors are, as it were, pressed out of the rectum, and swell in a very short time to an enormous size. They are of a much more vivid blood-red color, and will be found to be covered only by the lining membrane of the lower intestine. These are called "Internal Piles." The causes assigned for Hemorrhoids are many. People of sedentary habits are the subjects of them: costiveness, by the pressure of the hardened fœces on the veins, will produce them, and any thing that may irritate the rectum—for instance, a drastic purge, containing Aloes, Scammony, &c. Persons who never had Piles before taking Aloes and Scammony, have often been in such a state that they could hardly walk for them. Piles, no doubt, are, in some, constitutional, and hereditary, and, in such cases, the rectum is naturally weak. Persons annoyed with constipation, are the most likely to be afflicted with Piles; hence, free and intemperate livers, wine bibbers, feeble and relaxed constitutions, and those who take little exercise, pregnant women, and women who have borne many children, are exceedingly subject to them.

The treatment of Piles is very simple if rightly proceeded with at the commencement of the complaint—the grand object being to prevent constipation. When they are external and there is no inflammation, laxatives, such as Castor Oil, Senna, and Manna, and Epsom Salts combined, taken internally, and astringents applied externally, as Gall Ointment, or a decoction of White-Oak bark. The warm bath is an excellent adjunct to the cure of incipient Piles. In some cases it has been recommended to puncture the pile with the point of a lancet, and press out its contents, but this *should be done very cautiously*, for fear of hemorrhage. In chronic piles, the confection of Black Pepper has been of great service, if continued for some time. It appears to stimulate and give a new action to the parts. If there is considerable inflammation apply leeches upon them, or to the verge of the anus, using an evaporating lotion, a poultice, an opium injection, or an Opium Ointment, as the case may require, repeating these remedies as often as they may be necessary. The diet is of very great importance; it should be bland--Gruel, Mush and Molasses, Arrowroot & Rye soft cake with Molasses are the best articles of food. Fruits should be eaten freely—wine and exhilarating stimulants should be avoided, and as much outdoor exercise taken as possible.

An excellent plan is, also, to inject half a pint or more of cold water up the rectum every morning and suffer it to remain if possible twenty or thirty minutes. The following is useful as an Ointment:

Take one ounce of finely powdered Galls and seven ounces fresh Lard, and mix well together.

COMPOUND GALL OINTMENT,
FOR IRRITABLE PILES.

Take two drachms, finely powdered Galls, two ounces fresh Lard, one half drachm Solid Opium; powdered, one half a drachm British Oil; mix thoroughly and apply.

FOR CHILBLAINS.

Take one drachm rectified Spirits Turpentine, fifteen grains Sulp. Acid, two and a half drachms

Olive Oil; mix together and rub the chilblains night and morning, if they are unbroken.

POISONS AND THEIR ANTIDOTES.

This article is mainly taken, by permission, from a very valuable and comprehensive "Chart of Poisons and their Antidotes," by Dr. Thos. R. Crosby, of Hanover, N. H.

The following are some of the more common articles of poison by which human life is endangered or destroyed, either by accident or design, together with the symptoms attending their use, and the articles and measures which may be used to destroy their effects, and save life.

ALCOHOL.

Symptoms—Confusion of thought, inability to walk or stand, dizziness, stupor, highly flushed or pale face, noisy breathing.

Treatment—Excite vomiting by large draughts of warm water, by tickling the throat and by emetics; use stomach pump, pour cold water on head and back of the neck, keep up motion; whip the skin, palms of the hands, and soles of the feet with small cords or rods; give strong stimulants, as ammonia.

AMMONIA.

Symptoms—Strong acrid and burning taste in the mouth, heat in the throat and stomach, nausea, vomiting, great prostration, cold, clammy skin, small, frequent pulse.

Treatment—Antidote, Vinegar and Water, or any dilute, vegetable acid. Excite vomiting; give mucilages, emetics, cathartics, clysters, opiates.

AQUAFORTIS.

Symptoms—Lips, mouth and throat of yellow color; pain, burning and strangulation in swallowing; retching, vomiting of dark colored fluids, with shreds of mucous membrane, swelling of the throat; difficulty of swallowing and breathing, skin cold and clammy, pulse quick and small.

Treatment—Calcined Magnesia, Carbonate of Magnesia, chalk or whiting in water, soap and water, ashes and water, milk, white of eggs, oil and mucilages. Perhaps use a stomach pump. If suffocation is threatened, open the windpipe.

ARSENIC.

Symptoms—Sickness, faintness, burning pain in the stomach, vomiting, excessive thirst, dryness, heat and tightness of the throat, diarrhœa, slow and intermitting pulse, palsy, lethargy, insensibility, convulsions, &c.

Treatment—Hydrated, sesqui-oxide of iron, emetics of three to five grains, of sulphate of copper, ten to fifteen grains of sulphate of zinc; ipecac, mustard-seed; tickle the throat with the finger or feather; whites of eggs, milk gruel, flax-seed tea, warm water largely, oil and lime-water, calcined magnesia; stomach-pump.

BISMUTH.

Symptoms—Metallic taste in the mouth, heat and dryness of the throat, severe burning heat in the stomach and bowels, violent vomiting, sometimes of bloody matter, profuse diarrhœa, pulse small, frequent and irregular, skin cold and clammy, respiration difficult, fainting, convulsions, &c.

Treatment—Large portions of milk, whites of eggs, oil; promote vomiting, by large draughts of sickening drinks, and by tickling the throat with the finger or a feather; use stomach pump.

BLISTERING FLIES.

Symptoms—Burning in the throat and difficulty of swallowing, violent pains in the stomach and bowels, nausea, vomiting of bloody mucus, pain in the loins, desire to void urine, and passage of bloody water with great pain.

Treatment—Emetics; copious draughts of warm water, milk, mucilaginous drinks, tickling the throat with the finger or a feather.

BLUE VITRIOL.

Symptoms—Strong metallic taste in the mouth, belching, violent vomiting, and purging, griping pains, cramps in the thighs and legs, frothing at the mouth, headache, giddiness, convulsions, insensibility, &c.

Treatment—Early vomiting, by large draughts of warm water, and by tickling the throat, strong coffee, milk, white of eggs, wheat-flour and water, mucilages; stomach-pump.

CARBONIC ACID GAS.

Found in wells, cellars, mines, &c., and largely given off in the burning of charcoal in close rooms.

Symptoms—Drowsiness, difficulty of respiration, suffocation, face swelled and more or less discolored, sensation of great weight in the head, vertigo, loss of muscular power and insensibility.

Treatment—Admission of fresh air, friction, especially over the lungs, artificial respiration, by inflating the lungs by the mouth or bellows, application of strong stimulants to the mouth and nose, cold water poured upon the head and back of the neck. If the body be cold, a warm bath.

COBALT.

Of importance from its extensive use as a Fly-poison, children having eaten it and thereby been poisoned.

Symptoms—Heat and pain in the throat and stomach, violent retching and vomiting, cold and clammy skin, small and frequent pulse, respiration hurried, anxious and difficult; diarrhœa.

Treatment—Give freely milk, whites of eggs,

wheat-flour and water, nauseating teas, mucilages, emetics, clysters.

CORROSIVE SUBLIMATE.

Carelessly made use of in many families, as a bedbug poison.

Symptoms—Strong metallic or coppery taste in the mouth; burning heat and constriction of the throat; severe pain in the stomach and bowels; violent vomiting and purging; countenance swollen and flushed, or anxious and pale; pulse small, frequent and irregular; skin cold and clammy; tongue white and shriveled, respiration difficult; fainting, convulsions and insensibility.

Treatment—Albumen, which is contained in the whites of eggs abundantly: wheat-flour in water liquid starch, milk, iron filings; excite vomiting early by large draughts of warm water; mustard seed, tickling the throat, and emetics; use stomach pump.

DEADLY NIGHTSHADE.

Children are sometimes poisoned by eating the berries, which have a sweetish taste.

Symptoms—Dryness and stricture of the throat, nausea, vertigo, dilated pupils, dimness of sight laughter, delirium, redness and swelling of the face, convulsions, general paralysis and insensibility.

Treatment—Emetics of sulphate of zinc (ten to fifteen grains), or copper (three to five grains); large purgatives and clysters; take vinegar and water or other vegetable acids, freely; bitter infusions, lime water; stomach-pump; cold water poured on the head, and strong stimulants.

FOOL'S PARSLEY.

Taken by mistake for common parsley.

Symptoms—Heat of throat, and thirst; oppression at the stomach; nausea, vomiting and occasionally purging; cold and moist skin; small and frequent pulse; headache, vertigo and delirium.

Treatment — Emetics of zinc or copper; warm water, milk, flax-seed or chamomile tea, &c.; purgatives, clysters, warm bath, stimulants and opiates.

FOX GLOVE.

Symptoms—Intermitting pulse, vertigo, indistinct vision, nausea, vomiting, hiccough, cold sweats, delirium, syncope and convulsion.

Treatment—Emetics followed by strong stimulants (brandy, ether, ammonia), opiates, counter irritation, mustard seed poultices or blisters to the pit of the stomach, cold affusions.

FUNGUSES.

Or poisonous Mushrooms (Fungi), taken by mistake for eatable mushrooms.

Symptoms—Pain in the stomach; nausea, vomiting and purging, great thirst, colic pains, cramp, convulsions, vertigo, delirium.

Treatment—Emetics, purgatives, mucilages, acid drinks, stimulants (Ether, Brandy, Ammonia), opiates, bitters.

HELLEBORE.

Indian Poke, sometimes used in a poisonous quantity as a dressing for a sore.

Symptoms—Violent vomiting and purging; bloody stools; great anxiety, tremors, vertigo, fainting, sinking of the pulse, cold sweats and convulsions.

Treatment— Excite speedy vomiting by large draughts of warm water, molasses and water, tickling the throat by the finger or a feather, and emetics give oily and mucilaginous drinks, oily purgatives and clysters, acids strong coffee, camphor and opium.

HEMLOCK, (poison.)

Symptoms—Dimness of sight, vertigo, delirium, swelling of the abdomen with pain, vomiting and purging.

Treatment—Emetics of sulphate of zinc or copper, assisted by copious draughts of warm water, milk, flax-seed tea, chamomile, &c.; stomach pump, pouring cold water on the head and back; stimulants and acids.

HENBANE.

Symptoms—Appearance of intoxication, sickness, stupor, dimness of sight, delirium, great dilation of the pupils, insensibility.

Treatment—Emetics, with strong stimulants, as sulphate of zinc or copper, tartar emetic or ipecac, with mustard-seed or cayenne; acid drinks, ammonia, brandy, ether, strong coffee, cold affusion; stomach-pump and stimulating the skin.

LIME.

Symptoms—Heat in throat and stomach, nausea, vomiting, pain in the stomach, violent colic pains, diarrhœa, sometimes constipation.

Treatment—Vinegar, lemon juice, or any vegetable acid freely; demulcent drinks, opiates, warm bath, &c.

LUNAR CAUSTIC.

Symptoms—Burning pain in the stomach, nausea, retching, vomiting; sometimes extreme purging, cold and clammy skin; small, frequent, and irregular pulse, respiration difficult; fainting, convulsions.

Treatment—Common Salt in solution, abundantly; warm water; irritation to the throat, emetics, warm bath, purgatives, opiates.

MEADOW SAFFRON.

Symptoms—Nausea, vomiting, pain in the stomach, griping pains in the bowels, with violent purging; cold sweats; small, frequent, and irregular pulse.

Treatment—Excite vomiting (if not already free enough) by the use of nauseating drinks, tickling the throat, and emetics, mucilages, opiates, with stimulants.

MONK'S HOOD.
SEE OPIUM.

Symptoms—Nausea, violent vomiting and purging; vertigo; cold sweats, delirium, convulsions.

Treatment—Excite vomiting (if not already free enough) by emetics, large quantities of warm water, molasses and water, milk, flax-seed and chamomile teas, &c., acid drinks, stimulants, brandy, ether, ammonia, opiates.

MOUNTAIN LAUREL.

Of great importance, as honey made from its flowers is poisonous, and birds which feed upon its buds in winter are likewise poisonous.

Symptoms—Giddiness, violent flushings of heat and cold; sickness at the stomach, with repeated vomiting and purging; delirium, frequent and weak pulse, extreme debility, profuse perspiration, convulsions.

Treatment—Emetics, mucilaginous and nauseating drinks, warm water or molasses and water, tickling the throat, purgatives, clysters, strong stimulants, ammonia, coffee, cold affusion; stomach-pump.

MURIATIC ACID.

Symptoms—Extreme irritation; burning and sense of stangulation in the swallowing; discharge of shreds of mucous membrane, swelling of the throat, difficulty of swallowing and breathing; skin cold and covered with clammy sweat; pulse quick and small; lining membrane of the mouth and throat partially destroyed.

Treatment—Carbonate of magnesia, calcined magnesia, chalk or whiting in water, soap and water, ashes and water, whites of eggs, milk, oil, &c. Plaster from the wall may be beaten down to a paste with water and given; carbonate of soda with barley-water, slippery elm. If suffocation is threatened, open the wind-pipe.

MURIATE OF BARYTES.

Symptoms—Pain, burning and weight in the stomach, vertigo, dimness of vision, ringing in the ears, pain in the head, throbbing in the temples, paralysis, convulsions.

Treatment—Epsom or Glauber's salts in solution, emetics, large draughts of warm water, tickling the throat, flax-seed tea, stomach-pump; opiates in large doses

MURIATE OF TIN.

Symptoms—Strong metallic (coppery) taste, sense of tightness in the throat, difficult respiration, violent vomiting, with cramp in the stomach, severe colic pains, with purging, cold, clammy skin, small frequent pulse, paralysis, convulsions.

Treatment—Milk, largely administered, emetics, large draughts of warm water, tickling the throat, hot cloths to the stomach and bowels, soothing and opiate clysters.

NITRE.

Sometimes taken by mistake for some other salt.

Symptoms—Intense pain in the stomach, nausea, vomiting, profuse purging, bloody stools, severe colic pains in the lower part of the bowels, difficult breathing, great prostration, fainting, convulsions.

Treatment—Flax-seed tea, barley-water, molasses

and water, tickling the throat, emetics, opiates, stimulants, brandy, ether, &c.

NITRATE OF SILVER.
(SEE LUNAR CAUSTIC.)

NITRIC ACID.
(SEE AQUAFORTIS.)

NUX VOMICA.

Symptoms—An extremely persistent bitter taste in the mouth, muscular spasms, great rigidity, limbs fixed and stretched out, jaws spasmodically shut, drowsiness. If the symptoms are prolonged, nausea, vomiting, difficulty of respiration, asphyxia.

Treatment—The Cannabis Indica (a variety of the Hemp plant) has been recommended as an antidote; emetics, to produce immediate vomiting; stomach pump; vinegar and other vegetable acids in water.

OIL OF CEDAR.

Symptoms—Heat in the stomach, followed immediately by convulsions, with frothing at the mouth, pulsation ceases early. The body is warm a long time after death.

Treatment—Vomiting to be excited early as possible by large draughts of warm water, and other nauseating drinks, by a large dose of ground mustard-seed, and tickling the throat; use the stomach pump as early as possible.

OIL OF RUE.

Symptoms—Dryness of mouth and throat, thirst, heat and pain in the stomach and bowels, headache and delirium.

Treatment—Vomiting to be excited as quickly as possible, by large draughts of warm water, and other nauseating drinks; by ground mustard-seed, tickling the throat, emetics, acids; stomach pump.

OIL OF SAVIN.

Symptoms—Headache, delirium, strong general excitement, acute pain in the stomach and bowels, nausea, vomiting and purging convulsions.

Treatment—Vomiting to be excited by copious draughts of warm water; mustard-seed; tickling the throat, and emetics of Sulphate of Zinc or Copper; acid drinks, mucilages; stomach pump.

OIL OF TANSY.

Symptoms—Heat in the stomach, followed immediately by convulsions, and frothing at the mouth: pulsation feeble and soon lost.

Treatment—Vomiting to be instantly excited by copious draughts of warm water and other nauseating drinks; mustard-seed; tickling the throat, Sulphate of Zinc or Copper, acid drinks, mucilages, stomach pump.

The body will remain warm for a long time: strong odor of the oil.

OIL OF TAR.

Symptoms—Speedy insensibility, laborious, rattling breathing, coldness of the extremities, contraction of the pupils, suffusion of the eye, feeble pulse.

Treatment—Vomiting to be instantly excited by copious draughts of warm water, &c.

OIL OF VITRIOL.

Symptoms—Extreme irritation, pain, burning, and sense of strangulation in the swallowing; retching, vomiting, discharge of dark colored fluids and shreds of membrane from the stomach; swelling of the throat; difficulty of swallowing and breathing; cold, clammy skin; quick and small pulse. The lining membrane of the mouth and throat are partially destroyed, and of a white color.

Treatment—Carbonate of magnesia, calcined magnesia, chalk or whiting, mixed with water, soap or ashes and water, lime from the plastered wall beat into a paste with water, whites of eggs, milk, oil; perhaps the stomach-pump, but with great care. If suffocation is threatened, open the windpipe.

OPIUM

Symptoms—Giddiness, drowsiness, stupor, insensibility; pulse at first quick and irregular aud breathing hurried; afterwards breathing is slow and noisy, and the pulse slow and full. In favorable cases there is early nausea and vomiting.

Treatment—Excite instant vomiting by mustard-seed, copious draughts of warm water, and tickling the throat; give sulphate of zinc (ten to fifteen grains), or copper (three to five); use the stomach-pump early. Give strong stimulants ether, brandy, ammonia, strong coffee and tea. Pour cold water on the head and back of the neck and whip the skin, the palms of the hands, and soles of the feet with small cords or rods.

OXALIC ACID.

Generally taken accidently from its resemblance to Epsom Salts.

Symptoms—Hot, burning taste in the swallowing, immediate and constant vomiting, the matter thrown up being of a greenish or brownish color, and extremely acid; sometimes severe pain; collapse; pulse small, irregular and scarcely perceptible; numbness and spasms.

Treatment—carbonate of magnesia, calcined magnesia, chalk or whiting made into a cream with water and administered freely; lime-water with oil; emetics, mucilages; stomach-pump.

PHOSPHORUS.

Symptoms—Hot taste of garlic or onions in the

mouth; violent pains in the stomach; nausea, and vomiting, followed by great excitement of the arterial vessels; convulsions.

Treatment—Fill up the stomach with magnesia and water; give emetics and nauseating drinks to keep up the vomiting.

POPPIES,
(SEE OPIUM.)

POTASH.

Symptoms—Strong acid taste in the mouth; burning heat in the throat and stomach; sometimes vomiting and purging, with colic pains; cold, clammy skin; small, frequent pulse.

Treatment—Vegetable acids, vinegar, lemon juice or tartaric acid in water; emetics, clysters, opiates.

PRUSSIC ACID.

Symptoms—Instant sensation of weight and pain in the head; nausea, quick pulse. In large doses, instant insensibility, stupor, convulsions; loss of pulsation, slow and convulsive breathing.

Treatment—Application of strong ammonia to the nostrils; stimulating liniments to the chest; cold water poured upon the head and spine; chlorine Gas; a dilute solution of chloride of soda or lime.

POISON IVY

A running vine which is found covering walls, shrubs, trees, and in meadows.

This plant, by contact, and upon many without contact, produces violent erysipelatous inflammation, particularly with the face and hands. The symptoms are itching, redness, burning, swelling, watery blisters, and subsequently peeling of the skin. These effects are experienced soon after exposure, and usually begin to decline within a week.

Treatment—A light, cooling diet, an occasional purgative dose of Salts, and the application to the eruption of a weak solution of Sugar of Lead, or Green Vitriol. If the inflammation is severe, apply a soft poultice of cracker and milk, or of Slippery-elm bark, or still better, a decoction of Witch Hazel bark.

POISON DOGWOOD.

A small but beautiful shrub or tree, from ten to fifteen feet high, having a dark gray bark; its smaller branches of a lighter color, and its extreme twigs red. Its effects are similar to those of Poison Ivy, but more powerful.

The poisonous principle is most energetic during the burning of the wood. Symptoms and treatment the same as for the Ivy.

POISONOUS BITES.

Apply a ligature between the wound and the heart, to check the circulation, and then suck the wound thoroughly, taking care that there is no sore or broken skin in the mouth. A better plan is to cut out the bitten part freely, bathe it in warm water, and suck the wound, a ligature being applied as before. Apply a cupping-glass over the wound for a few minutes; remove it, cut out the wound, and apply again.

The system should be supported by administering the strongest stimulants, such as hot brandy and water, ammonia or ether. If no vomiting should occur, give a mustard emetic. If there be too much vomiting, give opium, and apply a mustard poultice to the pit of the stomach.

SALT OF SORREL,
(SEE OXALIC ACID.)

STRAMONIUM,
(SEE THORN APPLE.)

STRYCHNIA,
(SEE NUX VOMICA.)

SULPHATE OF COPPER,
(SEE BLUE VITRIOL.)

SULPHATE OF ZINC,
(SEE WHITE VITRIOL.)

SULPHURIC ACID,
(SEE OIL OF VITRIOL.)

SUGAR OF LEAD.

Symptoms—A burning, prickling sensation in the throat, with dryness and thirst; uneasiness at the pit of the stomach; nausea, vomiting; colic pains, constipation of the bowels, cold skin, feeble and irregular pulse, great prostration of the strength, cramps, numbness, paralysis, giddiness, torpor, insensibility.

Treatment—Epsom or glauber salts, (sulphates of magnesia and soda,) mucilages, milk, whites of eggs, wheat-flour with water, emetics; stomach-pump.

TARTAR EMETIC.

Symptoms—Nausea, severe vomiting, hiccough, burning heat and pain in the stomach; colic pains, violent purging, small, frequent and hard pulse; cramps, vertigo, fainting, and great prostration.

Treatment—Tea made of Oak bark, or Peruvian bark, strong green tea, mucilages, warm drinks, opium, opiate clysters.

THORN APPLE.

Symptoms—Vertigo, delirium, stupor, convulsions, paralysis, cold sweats, feeble and irregular pulse.

Treatment—Emetics of Sulphate of Zinc or Copper, mustard-seed, tickling the throat; stomach-pump.

TOBACCO.

Symptoms—Severe nausea, vomiting, headache,

sudden sinking of the strength, cold sweats, convulsions.

Treatment—Emetics, copious draughts of water, tickling the throat with the finger or a feather; purgatives, acid drinks, stimulants, brandy, camphor, &c.

VERDIGRIS,
(SEE BLUE VITRIOL.)

WHITE VITRIOL.

Symptoms—Bitter taste in the mouth, with sensation of choking; nausea and severe vomiting; pain in the stomach and bowels, purging, difficult breathing, quick and small pulse; coldness of the extremities.

Treatment—Albumen, whites of eggs, wheat-flour and water, milk abundantly, infusions of tea, oak bark, &c.; emetics, purgatives, and opiate clysters.

WHITE LEAD,
(SEE SUGAR OF LEAD.)

WOLF'S-BANE,
(SEE MONK'S-HOOD.)

MUSTARD EMETIC.

For an Adult, take one large tea-spoonful of ground mustard; put it in a little water. If it does not operate in fifteen minutes, the dose should be repeated.

LINIMENT FOR NEURALGIA.

Take two ounces Olive Oil, one half once Tinct. Opium, one half ounce Tinct. Aconite, one half ounce Aqua Ammonia. Mix well and apply to the part affected.

PILLS FOR NEURALGIA.

Take eighteen grains Ext. Conium, nine grains Ext. Belladona, twelve grains pulv. Ipecac, eighteen grains Aloes. Mix and make twenty-four Pills.

Dose: *One Pill* two or three times a day.

FOR COSTIVENESS.

Take 4 ounces of Figs, 2 ounces of Senna; chop them fine, and add Molasses; stir the mixture thoroughly; take a lump the size of a walnut at bed-time.

MUCILAGES.

The best and most common mucilages are Gum Arabic, Slippery-Elm bark, Cumfrey-root, with water, and flax-seed tea.

AN EXCELLENT TOOTH POWDER.

Take two ounces of Gum Myrrh, four ounces of Marsh Rosemary, one ounce Bole Ammonia, two ounces Orris root, four ounces Peruvian bark, two ounces refined Sugar, one ounce Castile Soap. Pulverise these very fine and mix.

COLOGNE WATER.

Take one half ounce Oil of Lavender, one half ounce Oil of Lemon, one ounce Oil of Rosemary, one ounce Oil of Bergamot, thirty drops Oil of Cinnamon, thirty drops Oil of Cloves, and one drachm Tincture Musk. Mix the whole in four pints of Alcohol.

COLOGNE WATER.

Take one and three fourths ounces Oil of Lemon, one and one eighth ounces Oil of Lavender, one and one eighth ounces Oil of Bergamot, one drachm Neroli. Mix the whole in one Gallon Alcohol, and keep in a cool place.

TONIC BITTERS.

Take one drachm Angustura bark, one half ounce Cinchona, two drachms Cardamon seeds, one drachm Elixir Vitriol, and twenty ounces pure water.

Dose :—*One table-spoonful* two or three times a day.

TINCTURES.

Tinctures are prepared by grinding or bruising the roots, leaves, or barks used, to a coarse powder, placing it in a proper quantity of clear or diluted Alcohol, letting it stand from seven to fourteen days, shaking each day.

INFUSIONS.

Infusions are generally obtained by pouring boiling water upon the substance, and letting it stand till it cools. When a more prolonged application of heat is desired, the vessel may stand for a while by the fire, but must not be permitted to boil. The vessel should usually be covered.

MATERIA MEDICA.

We give here a tolerably full list of the medical articles used in every family, together with their properties and usual effects upon the system.

GOLDEN THREAD—Tonic, promotes digestion, good in Dyspepsia.

HORSE RADISH—Highly stimulant, promotes secretion of urine.

CELADINE—Good in Jaundice, and for Ringworms and Warts.

MARSHMALLOWS—Emolient and soothing.

INDIAN TURNIP, or Dragon Root—Good for Colic, Coughs, Pain in the Breast, and Asthma.

BURDOCK—Alterative, excellent to purify the blood.

ARCHANGEL—A powerful stimulant, good for nervous Headache and trembling of the limbs.

MAYWEED—Good for Spasms, and to remove pain, and for derangement of the digestive organs.

PLEURISY ROOT—Promotes perspiration, removes wind, anti-spasmodic.

RED RASPBERRY—Good for Dysentery, Diarrhœa,

THE METHOD OF USING.

and to remove Canker from the mouth and throat.

Owen's Root—Good for Consumption, in first stages, general debility, Asthma and Sore Throat.

Thoroughwort—Valuable sudorific. Tonic, Alterative, Antiseptic, Cathartic, Emetic, Febrifuge, Diuretic, and Stimulant, one of the best of all Indian remedies.

Hardhack—Tonic and Astringent, good for weak state of the Stomach.

Catnip—Useful to produce perspiration.

Peppermint—Good to prevent vomiting, and for spasmodic pains in the Stomach.

Hoarhound—Very good in Coughs, Colds and all consumptive complaints.

Bayberry—Good to produce sleep, and remove pain.

Dandelion—Good in morbid state of the Liver.

Poplar Bark—Valuable in Dyspepsia, Asthma, and night Sweats.

Skunk Cabbage—Expectorant, good to allay spasms and to produce sleep.

Elecampane—Good for diseases of the Chest, and weakness of the digestive organs.

Butternut—A mild cathartic, good in Costiveness.

Liverwort—Used in Fevers, Liver Complaint, and Bleeding at the Lungs.

Hops—Tonic, good for nervous tremors, and to produce quietness or sleep.

Golden Seal—Tonic, Bracing, Cathartic, and used by the Indians in cases of Inflammation of the eyes.

Blood Root—Good for cleansing Ulcers, and Sores, excellent in Coughs and Croup, and in Catarrh.

Bitter Sweet—Good for chronic Rheumatism, and for Liver Complaint.

Mandrake—A sure and certain carthartic, also good for chronic affections of the Liver.

Hemlock—A powerful astringent, good for falling of the bowels.

Pitch Pine—Stimulant, good for suppression of the urine, and also good to expel worms.

Jerusalem Oak—One of the best Indian remedies for expelling worms.

Black Alder—Goo for bleeding at the lungs.

THE METHOD OF USING. 93

FIR BALSAM—Healing, good for fresh wounds and for weak stomach.

GENTIAN—Valuable Tonic; invigorating; good for general Debility and Gout.

SOLOMON'S SEAL—Good in female difficulties.

SAFFRON—Stimulant, and good to produce perspiration, and for Measles.

SPIKENARD—The Indians make great use of it in cases of sores, and ulcers—good for colds and coughs.

YELLOW DOCK—This is physical and bracing, and will evacuate the bowels without weakening the system.

WILD CHERRY—Tonic and invigorating, good in nervous debility.

WORMWOOD—Useful to correct the stomach, to give an appetite, and to break up a cold.

SCULL CAP—Tonic, Nervine, and Anti-Spasmodic.

MULLEN—Good in Dysentery and Piles, and for poultices.

PENNYROYAL—Stimulant and produces perspiration.

ELDER BERRIES—A gentle laxative, and tend to purify the blood.

PRICKLY ASH—Stimulant, Tonic and Energetic.

SLIPPERY ELM—Good for inflammations, external or internal.

SAGE—Good for Worms, and also for a gargle.

SARSAPARILLA—For purifying the blood—for chronic diseases of the liver or skin.

MUSTARD—Stimulant, good for emetics, and for Poultices.

WHITE OAK BARK—Strengthening, and valuable as a wash.

SPEARMINT—Diuretic, good in cases of Gravel.

COLTSFOOT—Emollient, and slightly Tonic, used in Coughs, and Asthma.

CARAWAY—Good in cases of wind colic.

BUCKTHORN BRAKE—Used in Coughs, Diarrhœa and Dysentery, and as a Tonic.

BLACK COHOSH—Slightly narcotic, sedative and acts upon the nervous system, and is useful in palpitation of the heart.

BETHROOT—Astringent, Tonic, and useful in cases of bleeding from the lungs and kidneys.

BALM—Moderately Stimulant, and is useful to produce perspiration.

BALM OF GILEAD—Useful in affections of the kidneys, and for Rheumatism.

PIPSISSEWA, OR PRINCE'S PINE—Tonic, Diuretic, and Astringent, useful in Dropsy, and diseases of the kidneys and bladder.

QUEEN OF THE MEADOW, OR TRUMPET WEED—Diuretic, Tonic, and Stimulant, good in diseases of the urinary organs.

RED ROOT, OR WILD SNOW BALL—Sedative, Astringent and Expectorant.

YARROW—Tonic, Astringent, and Alterative, good in bleeding from the lungs, and chronic Dysentery.

LOVAGE OR MAN OF THE EARTH—Good to expel humors of the blood.

VERVAIN—Good for Scrofula, Gravel, Coughs, and to expel worms.

MUGWORT—Valuable to expel worms.

VALERIAN—Useful in nervous complaints.

GOLDEN ROD—Gently laxative.

MOTHERWORT—Nervine, useful in Liver complaints.

CANKER ROOT—A sovereign remedy for Canker.

PLANTAIN—Good for expelling poisons.

Indian Wickerby—Good as a poultice for inflammation.

Life Root, or Ragwort—Diuretic and Tonic, valuable as a remedy in Gravel.

Indian Hemp—Powerfully emetic, and is also Diuretic, and Diaphoretic.

Ginseng—A mild Tonic, and Stimulant—good for nervous debility, and weak stomach.

Rock Rose, or Frostweed—Tonic, Astringent and Alterative, and good in Scrofula.

Culver's Root, or Blackroot—Tonic and laxative, a valuable remedy in affections of the liver.

Crawley—Good in inflammatory diseases, Cramps and night sweats.

Sumach—A good drink, good to wash and gargle the throat in ulceration.

Rhubarb—A thorough Cathartic.

Snakeroot—Good in Asthma, Coughs and Catarrh.

Blackberry—Good for Dysentery, and all bowel complaints.

Poke—Emetic, Purgative and produces sleep, good for nervous difficulties.

EXPLANATION OF TERMS USED IN THIS WORK.

Alterative—That which will restore healthy action gradually.

Astringent—Medicines which will draw up surfaces with which they come in contact.

Antidote—An opposing medicine.

Anodyne—A medicine which produces sleep and soothes pain.

Antiseptic—That which will prevent putrefaction.

Aromatic—Fragrant and spicy drugs, used to prevent griping of drastic purgatives.

Abdomen—Lower front part of the body.

Acrid—Irritating or biting.

Adult—A person of full growth.

Alkaline—Having the properties of an alkali.

Aqua Ammonia—Water of Ammonia.

Balm—Aromatic and fragrant medicine.

Balsam—Resinous substances possessing healing properties.

Bilious—An undue amount of bile.

Bowels—The intestines.

Capsicum—Cayenne Pepper.

Catarrh—Flow of mucus.

Cathartic—An active purgative.

Caustic—A corroding or destroying substance.

Chronic—Of long standing.

Constipation—Costiveness.

Contagious—That which may be given to another by contact.

Congestion—Accumulation of blood in a certain part.

Decoction—That which is prepared by boiling.

Diarrhœa—Looseness of the bowels.

Digest—To convert food into chyme; to prepare medicine with gentle heat.

Diuretic—That which increases the amount of urine.

Diluted—Reduced with water.

Drachm—Sixty grains, or a tea-spoonful.

Dyspepsia—Difficult, or bad digestion.

Elixir—A tincture prepared with more than one article.

Emetic—A medicine which produces vomiting.

Emollients—Softening and screening medicines.

Extremity—Applied to the Limbs.

Eruption—Pimple or blotch on the skin.

Evacuation—To discharge by stool, to haste away.

Evaporation—The act or process of escaping in the form of vapor.

Excretion—That which is thrown off—become useless.

Expectorants—That which produces or aids a discharge of mucus.

Extract—To take out an active principle from vegetables.

Express—To press out juices.

Excresence—An unnatural growth.

Felon—An abscess on the finger.

Filter—To strain through paper made for that purpose.

Flabby—Loose and soft to the touch.

Flatulence—Gas in the stomach.

Friction—Rubbing with the dry hand.

Formula—Medical prescription.

Function—The particular action of an organ.

Fistula—An ulcer.

Febrifuge—Medicine to drive away fever.
Fibre—A small thread-like substance.
Gallic Acid—An acid from the nut-gall.
Gostric—Belonging to the stomach.
Gentian—A root possessing tonic properties.
Gout—Inflammation of the joints of the toes.
Gravel—Crystaline particles in the urine.
Griping—A grinding pain in the stomach.
Gutta Percha—Dried juice of a certain tree.
Gutteral—Relating to the throat.
Gelatine—Isinglass.
Gaseous—Having the nature of gas.
Humors—The fluids of the body.
Hemorrhoids—Piles, bleeding piles.
Hygiene—Preserving the health by diet.
Immerse—To plunge under water.
Imbecile—One of weak mind.
Imbibe—To absorb—to drink.
Incontinence—Not being able to hold.
Indication—That which shows what ought to be done.
Indigenous—Produced naturally in a country.
Indigestion—Dyspepsia.

Indolent—Slow in progress, applied to ulcers, &c.
Infirmary—Where medicines are distributed.
Inflammation—Attended with heat and redness.
Infectious—Communicable from one to another.
Influenza—A disease of the nostrils and throat.
Infusion—Prepared by *steeping* in water, not boiling.
Ingredient—Each article of a compound mixture.
Inhalation—Drawing in the breath.
Injection—A preparation to be introduced by the rectum.
Internal—Upon the inside.
Jaundice—A disease caused by the inactivity of the liver.
Laxative—A very gentle cathartic.
Liniment—A fluid preparation, to be applied by friction.
Lotion—A preparation for a wash.
Macerate—To steep, to soften by soaking.
Malaria—Bad gases, supposed to arise from decaying matter.
Malignant—Pestilential and generally dangerous.
Mastication—The act of chewing.

Medical—Relating to medicine.
Membrane—A thin lining or covering—skin-like.
Morbid—Inactive and unhealthy,
Mucilage—A watery solution of gum.
Myrrh—A resinous gum.
Narcotic—Stupefying medicines, producing sleep.
Nausea—Sickness of the stomach, vomiting.
Nervous—Easily excited.
Nervine—That which will soothe nervous excitement.
Neuralgia—Pain in the nerves.
Nitre—Saltpetre.
Normal—In a natural and healthy condition.
Nostrum—A secret medical preparation.
Nutritious—Nourishing.
Organic—Pertaining to an organ or member.
Oxygen—One of the elements of the air.
Palliative—Affording relief.
Palpitation—Unnatural beating of the heart.
Paralysis—A loss of motion.
Pulmonary—Relating to the lungs.
Purgative—A gentle cathartic.
Regimen—Regulation of diet and habits.

Rash—A redness of the skin in patches.
Sanative—A curative medicine.
Sedative—The opposite of stimulation.
Specific—A remedy having uniform action.
Stitch—A spasmodic pain.
Symptom—A sign of disease.
Sudorific—Sweat-producing.
Tumor—An enlargement of a certain part.
Tonsils—The glands on each side of the throat.
Translation—Disease going to some other organ.
Vermifuge—Having the property to destroy worms.
Yeast—The principal of fermentation.

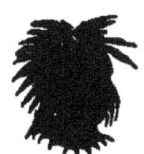

www.ingramcontent.com/pod-product-compliance
Lightning Source LLC
Chambersburg PA
CBHW031419160426
43196CB00008B/995